CONTENTS

I0423064

Bone Broth

What They Aren't Telling You About Bone Broths & Must Know Rich Broth Recipes

Jennifer Sullivan

ISBN: 1541345797
ISBN-13: 978-1541345799

FREE GIFT

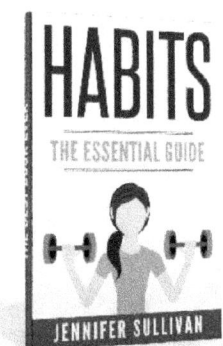

Discover The Secrets Behind How You Can Hardwire Your Brain For Success With Simple Habits!

Smoking, skipping breakfast, and procrastinating, these are some of the habits that we all know we should change and erase from our lives. However, even if changing these habits have been a part of your resolution list for so many New Years', it's still hard to let these habits go. Well, let me tell you that it is going to change now.

Not Everyone Wants To Admit It

To become the best you, you must stop looking at the big picture and start working on the small yet important stuff—your habits!

Visit my link to get your copy before the limited time promotion ends!...
https://cueballpublishing.leadpages.co/free-habits-ebook/

Introduction

I want to thank you and congratulate you for purchasing the book, *"Bone Broth: What They Aren't Telling You About Bone Broths & Must Know Rich Broth Recipes"*.

This book unveils the beautiful truth about bone broth and gives more than enough savory recipes to satisfy even the most skeptical minds.

No longer will you overlook this aspect of your cooking as its healthy qualities and enriching effects become more apparent. In the chapters following you will learn about bone broth's place throughout history, the nutritional breakdown as told by the experts, and also extra added tips and recipes to incorporate bone broth into!

Thanks again for purchasing this book. Enjoy!

From Ancient Times Back To Today

The origin of bone broth dates centuries back. If we talk about the era of the Stone Age, bone broth has been a vital part of human diet. It used to be taken as a delicious drink to have on a wintery night or given it to the sick ones to cure their cold.

A little modification added to the concept, the next thing you know, that bone broth has been transformed into a luxury soup. If we move forward in the roadmap of history, the early rest stops and certain restaurants had stocks and broths into their menus for the travelers to calm themselves from a cold night or a stressful journey.

With time, the use of bone broth took the shape of more of a cultural manifest due to its importance and benefits. Japanese have pork broth, Maldives having tuna broth, Koreans with beef bone broth, etc. Different cultures had different preferences.

With the passage of time, not only had it been treated as a meal to the people, but it was also used as a medicine by many healers. Bone broth was given as a medicine to the patients when nothing else worked to give them strength and overcome diseases.

In Chinese history, bone broth was used to increase blood in the body, strengthen the kidneys, and support a healthy digestive system. It was present in all Chinese clinics due to its excessive use in medical practices. In the history of Egypt, the famous physician Moses Maimonides was persistent in prescribing bone broths to his patients for colds and asthma in the early 12th century. In the Jewish history, it was known as "Jewish Penicillin" for the excessive use in medicine.

Along with all its medicinal importance in different cultures, the French society used to give bone broth to their army personnel regularly for their strength and fitness. In the 16th century, this broth was distributed to the homeless people of Paris and other areas to cover their nutritional needs.

The above-mentioned history has not been experienced by widely by the recent generation. Let's talk about the history that we actually remember. Our parents and grandparents used to prepare us bone broth when we were sick. They say it is their secret recipe that will magically take our illness away. With a simple recipe at home, parents still give their children broth in times of sickness. It was considered grandma's recipe.

I still get the recommendation of having the bone broth by my mom whenever I'm sick. But now, as the times are changing, its benefits and flavors are strikingly being recognized and bone broth has also been added to the finest dining restaurant's menu list. It is a renowned drink to every part of the culinary world. It would be wrong to consider the broth as only a warm drink. According to many chefs, food will lose its taste if the broth is eliminated from their cooking domain. Bone broths are used in many dishes to add distinct flavors into them as it enhances the taste and supplements the nutritional value.

With the rise in the Paleo diet and the dubiety towards gluten, bone broth did indeed attract the people who would like to follow a clean and healthy diet and also the ones who doubt the true benefits of our usual regimen.

Paleo diet greatly emphasizes the use of bone broth into routine. For one reason, it is very cheap and most importantly it has great healing power.

Regular use of bone broth cleans the stomach from the inside and brings in new life, qualities that are almost fictional to the modern diet.

Normally, bone broth and stocks are used interchangeably, considering them as one of the same. On the outside, they are pretty much the same, but its process in the back of the kitchen is a bit different. The only difference between the two lies in the concentration of bones with meat and the total cooking time.

A **broth** is an extract of meat with a few bones in the mixture, cooked for almost 2 hours or so, while a **stock** is a mixture of more bones extracts with some meat that is cooked for about 6 hours.

Now, bone broth is a combination of both a broth and the stock. The base of the bone broth is stock-like having bones and sometimes with their attached meat. It is cooked for more than 24 hours to extract the gelatin, potassium, magnesium, calcium and other minerals.

Slow and prolonged cooking causes the bones to become brittle at the end of the cooking. At the end, solid particles are extracted from the main mixture and relished like a broth. Top quality bone broths require bones from grass fed animals or wild fish. The purpose is to obtain bones from organic and honestly raised animals whose bones contain vitality and health.

Growth In Popularity

Within recent years bone broth has blown into the spotlight as no longer a backstage spectator in the health world. Even though some may treat it as a fad, there is no denying that such praise was much overdue! You and other folk who know the true power of bone broth can relish in the knowledge that it is not JUST a fad and can add positive changes to your life for years to come.

We can see around us the changes that others are making as well, either it being because of the 'fad' or if they truly know the benefits, we can still take advantage of the wider availability! News sources have covered the sprouting restaurants/bars that are basing their model around hearty and rich bone broths. It sounds like an alternate reality but there are really places growing in large cities in New York and California that give out warm cups of delicious broth like an awry coffee shop.

If one of these bars is by you, take pride in that true gelatin rich, nutrient dense bone broth is even easier to obtain and consume!

It is not only bars that have been springing up, but also online stores that will ship you real bone broth and not the flavored water broth that you see all the time at your supermarkets. These stores range from chicken broth to beef broth with varying flavors to the broth and even bone broth delivered in milk like cartons for easy pouring and storing. Talk about the unexpected!

As knowledge comes to be accepted by the general populace, we also see these online stores and other bone broth specific bars to be centered around the highest quality bones, grass-fed, non GMO fed, etc. The bar for standard bone broth seems to be rising all around us which makes it easier for us consumers to find the highest possible quality broth for healing and cooking purposes.

And as a quick side note while I am on the topic of bone broth businesses appearing up, I have also come into contact with a catering businesses that focuses on bone broth parties! It really shows that people are inspired by this health revolution and taking up grassroots action to propel the movement further, to everyone's advantage.

Traditions Are Valuable

I don't have the exact reason why but it is undeniable that we have an innate desire to not believe the advice our parents will tell us. We are all mini rebels when it comes to the 'strange' ideas of our parents. But one of the great tragedies is the outsourcing of bone broths.

If we happened to have parents who would save up old chicken bones after a meal or ask the butcher for bones, we might have turned our noses at our weird parents with their embarrassing homeland traditions. But in the true irony, how embarrassing is it for us that we have shunned one of the most healthy foods for it being too barbaric.

When I say we have outsourced our bone broth, I mean that we never make it ourselves anymore and instead buy it premade at the supermarket. Many times this sad excuse for broth is so poor that they have to add in monosodium glutamate or yeast extract for flavor, which you can find in the ingredient listing.

It is no coincidence that many cultures around the world have come to the conclusion that bone broth is a main staple of their dishes and diets. The Weston A Price Foundation is a great source to learn about the traditional diets of those cultures that have existed for hundreds and hundreds of years.

Their research shows that even though their diets could be considered primitive to us with no processed foods and not much access to sugar and other things we have wide availability to us today, they are notably more healthy and happier than many in the modern world on the modern diet!

Bone broth was not only a beneficial food for them, but it was also of the ethos that no food should be wasted if they had control over it. If bones were known to be able to be made into a rich and nutrient dense gelatinous broth, why on Earth would you throw it away? It is essentially a food inside your food, like a gift after you have eaten the meat off the bone!

At risk of sounding like an old geezer who reminisces of the old days, I think that it still needs to be said! Bone broth was better in the old days when people made it themselves with real bones and had the pot simmering for hours to extract the true essence out of the bones. It's simply undeniable!

In just the past few decades we have become more conscious of the source and quality of our food and I believe this is really flipping the food industry on its head. Along with our outsourcing of bone broth, many have come to battle the outsourcing of meat itself, to favor the higher quality of locally raised meats. More and more people are willing to shell out more money for meat that was not raised in appalling conditions, fed unnatural grain, and injected to force abnormal growth and promote a stressful and dismal existence.

I believe in the next few decades we will see a new whole system in place because the consumers are making their statements today and are changing their demands in the supply-demand fine balance!

Modernization Has Phased Out Critical Foods

I could understand objection to the addition of real bone broth into your life if it was really something out of left field. But in reality we're all using broth already in our foods and cooking anyway, just the worst possible quality!

When we really begin to understand that WE hold the choice and responsibility of health in our hands, dramatic changes are to come. And it feels even better when we know that slight tweak like using real homemade bone broth can boost your health in almost all aspects.

There's no doubt you've heard of the 'superfood' revolution. From my point of view, it seems a bit backwards of a movement. Does anyone else also notice that none of the superfoods are pills you can take or concentrated vitamins? Granted they are called super FOODS but the point still stands! People are putting more importance into the food they eat throughout the day instead of looking for the perfect modern quick chemical fix.

Even with all the advances in technology, it's hard to keep our body's intuitions at bay. Technology has still not mimicked basic foods that we used to eat and possibly end up altering our body in unknown ways in the long term. We thrive off of foods that are as close to the source as possible. This is also why the Paleo Diet has been gaining so much traction. Look for the least processed foods and eat only what our ancestors would have eaten.

My way of interpreting the current food revolution is that these foods shouldn't have the label 'superfoods.' To me, that makes it sound like they're found on the highest mountain and take some kind of magical alchemy to concoct! This couldn't be any further away from the concept of bone broth.

The bones can be gathered for free if you hunt around your local stores hard enough and the water itself to fill the pot (at least for now...) is also free! All added spices and vegetables are complimentary to the base, but even there you can use your veggie scraps. Once a large batch is made, it can be put in the fridge or freezer for anytime you want to spruce up a dish or want a quick warm glass of broth.

You can call it a 'superfood' if you want but to me it is more like my best friend when cooking! And also my alternative to a hot cup of tea in the morning.

Who Is To Blame For Sidelining Bone Broth?

It is never good to blame anyone for something that, in the end, is our own responsibility, but I believe I have a case for the reason things are the way they are so hear me out!

The resurgence of classic foods and knowledge about the source and quality of our foods show that we have taken our health into our own lives because we weren't explicitly taught correct nutrition and have been discouraged with the way things have been going. The place where most of us receive our dietary advice is the doctor, who admittedly has dangerously low expertise in nutrition.

So the trust in our doctors with regard to nutrition who are more educated in other health areas leads to a precarious result. Too many times I have heard of people going Paleo or talking about bone broth with their doctor and they have very little input on the idea or shun the health improvement and only recommend to 'take it slowly.'

I don't want to put words into doctor's mouths but much of their nutritional advice is outdated and that outdated information is what they tell their patients who have altered the supply-demand ecosystem of foods available for purchase.

Many promote the idea that vegetable oils are good for you when countless studies have shown the opposite and that the excess omega 6 fatty acids make us more unhealthy and sluggish. The one that kills me the most is that they demonize healthy fats in coconut oil and avocados, which are the best possible fats that you can ingest! Coconut oil has the highly praised lauric acid in its composition and is an incredible oil to cook with, as it remains stable during the high heat. I can go on about typical doctor lines of advice with counting calories, which adds extra life stress and weight, and the promotion of eating more carbs but I think you get my point.

I don't want you to start hating your doctor for misguiding you as they are definitely a great addition to our lives and wellbeing but you are warranted in feeling wary of their nutritional advice. If anything, it is good to hear their point of view and then research it further to see if it holds merit or if it simply something they have been saying since they left medical school decades ago.

Now more than ever we need to do our own research to come to a final conclusion as diets come and go, and on the surface they all seem like the true final diet you have been waiting for.

How To Make Classic Bone Broth

Step one is to… brace yourself… get some bones!

It can be as simple as keeping your chicken bones after a meal and piling them up until they can fit a pot but there are other potential options to get a free bone source.

In my experience, chain supermarkets that are branded like Whole Foods or Fairway always will put a price tag on bones, even if the bones were already in the garbage! Hopefully you will find a different result if you attempt to ask them for leftover bones in the meat sections. However, smaller butchers and fish markets seem to have no problem with giving you free bones.

For a few years I had a relationship with a local fish market man who allowed me to pick any and as many fish skeletons out of a bin after they have been filleted. Make sure you get yourself out there and become familiar and friendly with your local small shops that might have leftover bones lying around!

The only criteria I have is to find and prioritize the cartilaginous bones like chicken feet, beef knuckles, chicken necks, fish skeletons, etc. Other bones are not to be avoided as they would add flavor but for extraction of gelatin and the properties that make the broth feel full, cartilaginous bones are king!

My only warning is to avoid salmon and other oily fish when using fish carcasses as they throw a monkey wrench into the glory that is bone broth. When using carcasses from my fish market connect, I ended up using some salmon bones for one batch and the fisherman gave me a strange look and tried to warn me. Needless to say, I left the salmon bones in his bin every time afterwards!

Let's take a look at how to make a classic bone broth at home without any additional flavors. Bone broth can be used to make various dishes as it enhances the taste and flavors of meals.

Further recipes shall be discussed later, but right now we shall make the basic bone broth. It takes a day or two to make the bone broth with low heat. The equipment required is a pressure cooker or a general stockpot, and a fine mesh strainer or any filter.

Ingredients

- Chicken, beef, mutton or fish bones – 2 or 3 pounds

- Sea salt (optional) – 1 tsp.

- Black pepper – 1 tsp.

- Apple cider vinegar – 1 tbsp.

- Veggies like onions, carrots, capsicum, garlic, etc.

Directions

1. Roast the bones at 350F for half an hour if they have meat attached to it. The roasted meat adds a good flavor to the prepared broth.

2. Put the roasted bones into a cooker or a stockpot and add water into it. The bones must be dipped well in the poured water. Water must be cold or room temperature.

3. Add black pepper and salt into it. Salt is optional because the bones themselves release sodium in such a manner that it covers up for salt requirements.

4. Add apple cider or normal vinegar into the pot.

5. Vegetables are optional. 1 large roughly chopped onion, 1 or 2 carrots, ½ capsicums, or any other vegetables desired can be added.

6. Heat the mixture till boiling and then immediately bring it to a slow heat. It should be cooked slowly with open lid and continuous simmering. Skim off the foam of impurities that cover up the top surface of the broth.

7. Skimming can be done by a filter or mesh strainer.

8. Chicken bones are cooked for about 24 hours, while lamb or ox bones are cooked for 46 to 48 hours.

9. Seasoning can be done by adding parsley or herbs and cover up the lid for 15 minutes.

10. Filter the broth and pour it in a jar or any other container and cool it instantly to avoid any impurities from forming in the broth.

11. Your very own homemade bones broth has been prepared!

It can be consumed as it is on a daily use, or it can be used to prepare various delicious soups, stews and curries.

According To The Nutritionists

Bone broth has a great variety of nutritional value that has not only been recognized by the nutritionists, but also by chefs from around the world. More recently bone broth has become an important part of the Paleo diet.

Immunity

It is said that bone broth provides a certain level of immunity to the body. It also nourishes the damages done to the body due to certain injuries and diseases. That is why bone broth is often referred to as "Jewish Penicillin." This is why some nutritionists advise the consumption of bone broth to their patients who are recovering from illness or sufferings from a weakened disease.

The procedure of preparation for bone broth allows the bone marrow to get dissolved, that when consumed, the body builds both red and white blood cells, thus making the blood healthier. This healthier blood allows a stronger immune system in fighting off future infections. The art of longevity that is practiced by the Chinese includes the regular use of bone broth for healing and an overall strong body.

In the trending times, the use of bone broth has also become popular in the professional sports field as well. In the Washington Post, an ESPN report was provided highlighting the quick recovery of a high profile basketball player, Kobe Bryant, only by the daily use of bone broth. He had suffered from a ruptured Achilles tendon and a fractured knee. A quick recovery was seen followed by tremendous health after the use of bone broth soups.

It may seem over exaggerated but science approves of the mythical health benefits of bone broth. According to a famous wellness expert and a Chef Corinne Trang, bone broth has clear medicinal qualities. It is rich in minerals and is a supplemental source to the critically deficient population. Bone broth is one of the best options in making the body's blood healthier and the immune system stronger.

Reduce Joint Pain

Glycosaminoglycans (GAGs) are essential for our joint tissues. These are a series of connected tissues, which are also called collagen. The popularity of GAGs or collagen has been increased due to its benefits of skin and joint tissues.

Many people take supplements to cater for their nutritional values. But if any nutritionist is asked, all of them will prefer the use of natural ways of consuming collagen. Bone broth is rich in collagen that has its constructive impacts on joints of the body, which makes them stronger and prevents joint pain.

It has a visible effect in making healthier connective tissues, giving strength and support especially in old age.

Healthier Bones

Bone broth is, generally speaking, a good guy, the kind of guy who watches out for you when you're under the weather and helps you get back on your feet when your daily routine takes a bit too much out of you.

One of the best and probably the most obvious benefits of bone broth is its benefit for your… wait for it…bones…duh right? Most people have adopted taking supplements as a part of their daily ritual, following a trend that has swept the nation.

But what if you get whatever calcium, magnesium and phosphorous your body needs to keep its bones healthy and fit from a simple broth, a bone broth. Research has proven that a well-made bone broth contains almost all necessary minerals to keep your bones fit and in good working condition without the need for any artificial supplements.

Another less obvious benefit of bone broth is its effects on the growth of hair and nails. Bone broth contains naturally occurring proteins that our bodies seem to thrive on. These are often also found in very high-end hair treatments and products, which aim to promote general hair wellbeing and growth.

Bone broth however provides these proteins in a more natural manner without the need for processing and adding harmful chemicals to the end product or diluting its effects. The proteins are known to promote hair growth, improve overall hair health, and also improve the color and texture of your nails.

Stronger Teeth

Research says that the crucial portion of the bones used in making bone broth is the bone's calcium and potassium. The prolonged cooking extracts the mineral content from the bones and releases it into the final dish. Potassium and calcium are the major minerals that contribute to the teeth.

With more minerals consumed, it results in making our saliva healthier to be able to help in reducing the tooth decay. Saliva has a direct contact with the gums and teeth. Oral health is maintained through this nutrient rich saliva and healthier saliva helps in reviving healthy enamel on our weakened or affected teeth.

Since bone broth contains GAGs, oral health is likely to become improved, the connective tissues help in reinstating the infected gums. The gums that had been infected by 'bad bugs' and whose ligaments that have been nutritionally ignored are strengthened the bone broth collagen along with connective tissue in the mouth. These healthier tissues in return restore the ligaments in the gums that tighten the hold of teeth, making them stronger and healthier.

Furthermore, almost all doctors believe that diseases that manifest themselves in our body can be avoided through well-maintained oral health as the pathogens enter through our mouth or nose. This homemade solution seems to be more than meets the eye!

Complimentary Health Tips

Whether reason you are interested in bone broth or an overall health improvement, these extra tips can help keep your eye on the prize! When making a positive change in your life, it's not a bad idea to stack the odds in your favor. After all, you deserve to make it easier on yourself. Most come to the concept of bone broth benefits after being so tired of the current hand they've been dealt, knowing that more powerful truth is out there to find, but many also come from a health mindset who just want to make their body and life even more grand! It is for these common two reasons that this section is needed.

Success tips are rarely shared between people unless they are close friends yet everyone has small tidbits about small hacks that they have come to swear by! In a time of information encompassing books of all topics, it is easy to slip into a whirlwind of information and virtually come out with nothing! These are my tested main pillars to keep me focused, dedicated to my diet, and constantly waking up with a grin on my face! :)

Power Of Visualization

This might be the most 'woo woo' and 'hullabaloo' tip here but I cannot stress its importance enough! There is no denying, we are our thoughts.

You might not put the unconscious puzzle pieces together but everyday you are visualizing! You wake up and think about the day ahead of you, the work you have at your office left with the expectation of how to resume it. You look forward to lunch and visualize its impending arrival with thoughts of what you might order and visualizing how you expect it to taste. And with these thoughts, you imagine yourself acting in a specific manner that you have expected of yourself!

Now imagine that in all those situations you saw yourself as incredibly happy and committed to your new habits, and FELT it in your soul. Our naturally neutral daily visualization becomes a comfortable cycle that takes mental power to actually combat but the benefits can be astounding! I'm not saying that you can change the future you, but if you imagine yourself in settings you frequent with a radiance and happiness about you enough, you will see a clear difference.

How do you want to realistically be in the near future?

How do you want to look?

How do you want to feel and exude to others?

Really think about these questions and come to a clear answer. Then set apart a few minutes, preferably in the morning, close your eyes, and vividly see yourself and feel inside as you have wished. You will find that imagining your mental projection of yourself as happy is sometimes enough to put a smile on your face. We can strive all we want but a goal puts thing in perspective. Never underestimate the power of your mind!

Prioritize Positivity Over Negativity

I know, you're probably thinking, 'What an obvious topic! I know that already.' Of course we all avoid negativity… right?

Yes and No!

Like I mentioned in my Visualization section, we eventually let our minds run on autopilot, even if it's a neutral to destructive thought pattern and we also can become content with negative relationships. The only difference is that people can change on their own accord so it becomes our own responsibility to evaluate if they are still a positive addition to our life and passions. We know to avoid truly negative people who can be categorized as 'haters' or people who don't vibe with us anymore. This is the obvious negativity but the more sinister is slightly hidden.

We all know of that person as much as it hurts me to say it. The person who doesn't take your commitments seriously and brushes off changes you are implementing into your life to better yourself. The person who's passive aggressive about your changes and doesn't like that your life improvements make them guilty of their own lack of action.

Simply put, this person is not adding significant value into your life and you can bet that they aren't helping you stay motivated in any way. The worst part is that these people tend to be family or friends that you have known a long time; so taking drastic action in your relationship with them is incredibly painful.

If you want to mend the relationship for the both of you, confront them with your concerns. Hopefully, if they're a true friend, they will understand and possibly come around, but if all else fails you have to distance yourself from them. Having a positive network around you can greatly increase your chances in succeeding in all endeavors.

Hand pick your circle and watch the difficulty of staying on diet/task ease up significantly!

Add Extra Fun Into Your Life

It is truly a modern day tragedy that the word fun and fit are so often separated that the only thing they have in common is they both start with an 'f' and are three letter words!

To tell you the truth, I really hate the gym. Like really hate it. Even when I go with friends or family. But quickly I came to realize that I wasn't doomed into a pit of eternal lack of fitness! When framed in a different view, all it happened to be was a learning experience that showed me what I didn't like.

The idea of waking up hours earlier than normal to force a time slot before work was nothing but pure torture for me. But then I slowly started to experiment and find activities that I truly enjoyed, and immediately that had me more consistently active than my brief stint at the gym!

Many have no problem with a gym routine and find great results from it and I applaud them! But that's not me.

Regarding exercise, I find that less is more.

Like the New Year's Resolutions that fall to the wayside at an alarming rate, hard uncomfortable changes can only be stuck with for so long. Take it easy and go one step at a time!

Grab a few friends and go on a hike through a trail or up a local mountain. Join a ballroom dance class, head out ice-skating, or practice your swimming skills at the pool. Not only will making your 'work out' fun make you more likely to stick with it and lose weight, but also feel happier and look forward to each day!

If you can get friends in on the fun, it is almost impossible to stop the positive cycle! And when I say that less is more, I also mean that small activities add up. If you solidify these changes into a few times per week, it doesn't feel as burdensome and can help build momentum to keep the streak going!

Soon you will feel awkward if your momentum streak breaks. In my experience, the feeling is similar to when you're rushed to skip a daily ritual like brushing your teeth or skipping breakfast. The whole day just seems off and you feel compelled to jump back on the wagon!

Delicious Broth Recipes

There are various soups, stews, sauces and dishes made out of bone broths. Some of the dishes are especially used in Paleo diet and for weight watchers. The great news is that the dishes made out of bone broth are not only healthy but they are also very delicious in taste! I personally love bone broth recipes and I don't hesitate to incorporate them into my daily diet. The people, who like to have the food fresh, can freeze the bone broth beforehand and slowly consume, just as much broth needed in preparing broth recipes.

The major hard work is only the making of bone broth, the rest is very easy and less time consuming. All you will need to do is to bring out the broth from the freezer and follow these simple recipes to make delicious and healthy food. Serve it to your family and I assure you they will appreciate you for it! It's advised to all people who want to adopt a healthier diet to have bone broth in their kitchens for daily cooking. Whether you want to cook soups, stews or even sauces, just make them out of the bone broths instead of adding simple water into them.

Broth Soups

Broths most famously make soups of all kinds. Some people specifically have soup in cold weather or when sick. But it is a personal experience that having soup after a tiresome day or a stressful week actually really helps in sooth your tired body. Especially while watching a relaxing movie, a hot cup of soup really compliments the environment.

Apart from this, soups are mostly popular for starters. They aggravate our hunger and prepare us for dinner. Some of my personally tried soup recipes are provided in this section.

Chicken And Sweet Potato Soup

Servings: 4-5 servings

Ingredients:

- Olive oil – 2 tbsp.

- Salt – 2 tsp.

- Black pepper – 1 tsp.

- White pepper – ½ tsp.

- Onions – 1 medium sized, chopped finely

- Corns – 1 cup

- Sweet potatoes – 2 medium sized, cut nicely

- Celery – 3 ribs, chopped finely

- Thyme – ½ tsp.

- Lime (juice only) – 1 tbsp.

- Chicken broth (reduced sodium) – 4 cups

- Chicken breast (already cooked or boiled) – 2-3 pieces, sliced evenly into smaller ones

- Oyster sauce (optional) – ½ tsp.

- Corn flour (optional) – 2 tbsp.

Directions:

1. In a medium sized pot, add oil and onion. Fry it on a light-medium heat till the onions get light pink.

2. Add celery into it and fry till the vegies are light brown.

3. Add in it bone broth, sweet potatoes, thyme and lime. Bring the mixture to boil at a high heat.

4. Lower the heat to a medium one after reached boiling. Add chicken pieces and corns in it. Keep stirring it occasionally till the potatoes are tender and soft.

5. Add oyster sauce into the mixture to include a new flavor into the soup. Other sauces like soy sauce, vinegar and chili sauce are optional to make it spicy.

6. If a thicker soup is required, then mix the corn flour in a small quantity of water separately. Slowly add the corn flour mixture into the soup till the desired thickness is reached.

7. Serve it in cups and enjoy a healthy mixture of chicken and veggies.

Vietnamese Noodle Soup

Servings: 4-5 servings

Ingredients:

- Salt – ¾ tsp.

- Black peppercorns – ½ tsp.

- Ginger – 2cm stem, chopped

- Whole star anise – 3

- Cloves – ½ tsp.

- White onion – 1 large size

- Green onion – 4 diagonally cut

- Cinnamon – 1 stick

- Green or red chilies – 1-2 in number

- Capsicum – ½ or 1 medium size

- Corns, olives, mushrooms, kale, tomatoes, beans, or any other veggies for topping (optional)

- Fish sauce – 1 tbsp.

- Soy sauce – 3 tbsp.

- Lime juice – 1 tbsp.

- Water – 3 cups

- Beef broth – 4 cups

- Beef fillet steak – 50g chopped into small pieces, cooked or boiled

- Noodles – 12 Oz

Directions:

This recipe is easier to follow if it is broken down in 3 steps.

Step 1:

1. Pour the beef broth and water in the cooking pot and add in it salt, black peppercorns, cinnamon and ½ tsp. of white pepper (optional).

2. Add whole star anise, cloves, garlic, white onion, capsicum and red or green chilies.

3. Cook at high heat covering the top and let it simmer for about an hour or so.

4. Now uncover the top and strain the broth by a kitchen strainer into another container.

Step 2:

5. Separately boil the noodles in water. Add 1 tbsp. of oil and ½ tbsp. of salt in the water for boiling. This adds more flavor to the

noodles. Follow the noodle instructions from the packet for boiling.

6. Let aside the noodles to cool off for 5-10 minutes.

7. All these noodles into the initially made broth.

Step 3:

8. Mix soy sauce, lime and fish sauce in the broth solution. Stir well.

9. Add as many vegetables as you like. Corns, olives, mushrooms and sea weeds give good flavor to the noodle soup.

10. Add meatballs in the soup.

Vietnamese noodle soup is ready to be served.

Chicken Vegetable Soup

Serving: 4-5 Servings

Ingredients:

- Chicken broth – 6 cups

- Chicken boneless (chest) – 1 piece

- Capsicum – 2 medium size

- Carrots – 4 large size

- Green onions – 2 in number

- Lettuce – 2 small sized or 1 large

- Corn – ½ cup

- Egg – 1

- Corn flour – 2 tbsp.

- Salt – 1 tsp.

- Black pepper – ½ tsp.

- Vinegar – 2 tbsp.

- Soy sauce – 2 tbsp.

- Chili sauce – 1 tbsp.

Directions:

This recipe should be followed in two steps:

Step 1:

1. Pour the chicken broth in the cooking pot and add 1 capsicum, 2 carrots, 2 green onions, 1 lettuce and any other additional veggies that you'd like for the flavors. Save corn for the next step.

2. Cook at medium heat for 15 minutes till the vegetables completely allocate its flavor into the mixture. At this point, the vegetables are almost transparent.

3. Strain the soup and remove all the veggies from the solution. This is an additional step which brings rich veggie flavor and nutrition in the soup.

Step 2:

4. Now add all the vegetables again including 1 capsicum, 2 carrots, 1 lettuce and corn.

5. Add salt and black pepper.

6. Add sauces including vinegar, soy sauce and chili sauce.

7. Beat the egg separately and slowly add it in the soup while constantly stirring the mixture. In this way, egg is entirely mixed forming thin egg strands.

8. Separately make a corn flour solution by mixing the corn flour in a small amount of water. Slowly add the mixture in the soup while maintaining continuous stirring, till the desired thickness is maintained. If a loose soup is desired, corn flour is not needed in such a case.

9. Chicken vegetable soup is prepared and ready to be served!

Chicken Corn Soup

Servings: 4 servings

Ingredients:

- Olive oil – 2 tbsp.

- White pepper – ½ tsp.

- Black pepper – 1 tsp.

- Salt – to taste

- Sugar – 1 tsp.

- Chinese salt – ½ tsp.

- Eggs – 2

- Corn flour – 3 tbsp. dissolved in 3/4th cup broth

- Corns – 1 ½ cups

- Green onion – 1 cup, chopped finely

- Vinegar – 1 tsp.

- Soy sauce – 1 tsp.

- Chili sauce – 1 tsp.

- Bone Broth- 4 cups

- Boneless boiled chicken –

Directions:

1. Heat olive oil on a medium heat till it is hot.

2. Add chicken broth in the cooking pot. Bring it to boil.

3. Add sugar, white pepper, black pepper, salt and Chinese salt. Mix well.

4. Add boiled shredded chicken pieces in the soup.

5. Gradually add the corn flour mixture while stirring in one direction.

6. Cook the soup. When it comes to the first boil, add corns.

7. As the soup thickens, remove it from the heat. Slowly add the beaten eggs in a swirl and don't mix until the eggs are floating on the top. Mix till soft.

8. Put it back on fire. Once it comes to a boil, soup is ready.

9. Garnish it with chopped green onion. Serve hot.

Tomato Soup

Servings: 4-5 servings

Ingredients:

- Olive oil – 2 tbsp.

- Salt – 1 tsp. or as according to taste

- Black pepper – ½ tsp. or as according to taste

- Garlic – 2 cloves, chopped finely

- Tomato puree – 2 cups

- White onion – 1 medium to large size

- Bay leaf – 2 leaves

- Celery stick – 1, chopped in small pieces

- Corn flour – 1 tbsp. mixed in a little water to form paste

- Heavy cream – 2 tbsp.

- Bone broth – 2 cups

Directions:

1. Put oil in the cooking pan and heat it at a low flame.

2. Add garlic and onion in it. Fry them till the vegetables are slightly transparent.

3. Add bay leaves and celery stick. Cook for 2-3 minutes. Keep stirring so the veggies don't stick to the bottom.

4. Add tomato puree and bone broth in the pan.

5. Cook till a smooth solution is formed at a low or medium heat.

6. Add salt and pepper.

7. Add cream and sugar. Stir well.

8. Now add corn flour paste in the soup till the required thickness is formed. Keep stirring while pouring in the corn flour solution.

9. Top it with green onions or mushrooms to add more flavors.

10. Meatballs or boiled noodles can also be added into it.

11. Serve it hot. Enjoy!

Lentil Soup

Servings: 4 servings

Ingredients:

- Olive oil – 2 tbsp.

- Salt – 2 tsp.

- Black pepper – 1 tsp.

- White onion – 1 medium size, finely cut

- Carrots – 2 medium size chopped

- Tomatoes – 1 cup peeled and mashed

- Celery – ½ cup, chopped finely

- Oregano – 1 tsp.

- Dried basils – 1 tsp.

- Lentils – 2 cups, washed and rinsed

- Coriander – ½ tsp.

- Chicken broth – 8 cups

- Vinegar – 1 tbsp.

- Soy sauce – ½ tbsp.

Directions:

1. Heat the olive oil in the cooking pot at a medium heat till it's hot.

2. Add onion, garlic, carrots and celery in the oil. Fry for almost 2 minutes till the onions are tender and translucent.

3. Add salt and black pepper, and stir well.

4. Mix oregano, coriander and dried basil.

5. Add lentils and mix well.

6. Pour in chicken broth and tomatoes and cook well till it boils. Lower the heat and cook for 45 minutes or an hour till the lentils are tender and soft.

7. Add vinegar and soy sauce in the soup and taste your creation. If more salt needed, add more according to your taste.

8. Serve hot and enjoy!

Broth Sauces

Bone broths can be used in making various types of sauces. We have a few of them in this book; but if any other sauce is needed to be prepared, then the major trick is to replace water or any other liquid with bone broth. It will bring entirely new and more enjoyable flavors to the food.

Simple Broth White Sauce

Try this sauce with French fries. It is pure love!

Ingredients:

- Salt – 2-3 pinch of it

- Black pepper – 2-3 rounds

- All-purpose flour – 2 tbsp.

- Butter – 2 tbsp.

- Chicken broth – 1 cup

- Cheese (optional) – 1-2 slices

Directions:

1. Put butter in a pan at a low heat till it melts.

2. Add salt and black pepper.

3. Add all-purpose flour and stir constantly.

4. Mix bone broth in the pan and whisk till the solution is saucy and bubbly.

5. Add cheese and whisk till melted and mixed.

6. Serve immediately.

Chicken Broth Pasta Sauce

If the regular pasta sauce is made from bone broth, the flavors of the entire dish bring a restaurant-like experience to the regular homemade dish.

Servings: 4 servings

Ingredients:

- Olive oil – 2 tbsp.

- Garlic – 2 cloves, chopped finely

- White onion – 1 small sized

- Green onion – 2 regulars

- Additional vegetables like carrots, capsicum, lettuce, olives, etc

- Corn flour – 2 tbsp.

- Salt – 1 tsp.

- Cooked meat

- Cooked noodles

Directions:

1. Put olive oil in a pan and heat it at a low flame.

2. Fry white onion and garlic at medium flame till they get tender.

3. Lower the flame and add broth and mix corn flour solution.

4. Add salt and mix till the sauce is thick enough.

5. Add in vegetables and meat into it.

6. Add noodles and chopped green onions.

7. Sprinkle oregano in the end and serve.

Bolognese Sauce

Servings: 4 servings

Ingredients:

- Olive oil – 1 tbsp.

- Salt – to taste

- Black pepper- ½ tsp.

- Onions – 2 medium size

- Carrots – 2 medium size

- Tomatoes – 3 medium size

- Tomato puree – 3 or 4 tbsp.

- Mixed herbs (Basel, oregano, thyme, rosemary, etc) – 1 tsp.

- Green onion – 1 cup

- Garlic – 2 tbsp. crushed

- Mince – 500g

- Red chili – 1 finely chopped

- Bone broth – 1 cup

- Parmesan cheese (optional) – 60g

Directions:

1. In a heavy base saucepan, add olive oil at a medium heat.

2. Fry garlic, onion, carrots and green onions for 10 minutes. Stir often.

3. Once all the vegetables are soft, increase the heat to medium high and mix in the mince.

4. Once the mince is brown and caramelized, add tomatoes and tomato puree with the red chili.

5. Stir with a wooden spoon preferably. Mix in the broth.

6. Add herbs and season with the spices, cover the lid and lower the heat to the minimum.

7. Cook for an hour on low heat until the sauce is thickened and rich in flavor.

8. Once the Bolognese is almost finished cooking, add parmesan cheese off the heat.

9. Serve it with pasta or crusty bread!

Marinara Sauce

Marinara sauce is widely used in potato wedges, boiled or baked vegetables, lasagna, mutton chops, meat loafs, fried chicken, meat balls and spaghetti. It is a healthy yet delicious sauce.

Ingredients:

- Olive oil – 1 ½ tbsp.

- Salt – to taste

- Black pepper – to taste

- White onion – 1 cup finely chopped

- Grounded garlic – 1 ½ tsp.

- Green onion – ½ cup

- Tomato – 5, pureed

- Chicken broth – 1 cup

Directions:

1. Heat the olive oil in a large pan at a medium heat.

2. Sauté onion over medium heat until translucent.

3. Add garlic to the onions and cook for half a minute.

4. Mix in the broth over high heat until boiling.

5. Keep heating and mixing until the mixture is highly evaporating.

6. Add tomatoes, green onion, salt and pepper.

7. Cook on medium heat for 2 minutes. Cover the sauce and simmer on the lowest heat for 15-20 minutes.

8. Once the water is evaporated and the desirable thickness is obtained, take it off the heat.

9. Enjoy the sauce!

Light Alfredo Sauce

This sauce is very famous for its diverse use. It is used in a very versatile manner. It is topped over steaks, pasta, spaghetti, baked vegetables and even French fries. It's really hard to find anyone who wouldn't like Alfredo sauce.

Ingredients:

- Salt – to taste

- Chinese Salt – 1 tsp.

- Pepper – to taste

- Grounded red chili – ¼ tsp.

- Butter – 4 tbsp.

- All-purpose flour – 3 tbsp.

- Parmesan cheese (optional) – ½ cup

- Milk – 1 cup

- Broth – 2 ½ cups

Directions:

1. In a large sauce pan, preferably non-stick, melt butter into cream over low heat.

2. Add all-purpose flour into mixture and whisk until the flour is completely incorporated in the butter.

3. Once the flour comes to a creamy color or texture, take it off the heat.

4. Add milk and broth 1 cup at a time. Keep whisk it vigorously. Make sure there are no lumps.

5. Once all of the mixture is added, put it on the medium heat.

6. Add salt, black pepper, Chinese salt and grounded red chilies when the sauce is smooth.

7. Once the sauce reaches a desirable consistency, remove it from the heat and add cheese. Whisk till the cheese is melted.

8. Serve as a side to any food desired!

CONCLUSION

Thank you again for joining me on this journey!

I hope this book was able to help you learn more about the awesomeness that is bone broth and gave you some new awesome ideas to try out.

The next step is to grab that spoon and get to sipping!

Finally, if you enjoyed this book, then I'd like to ask you for a favor, would you be kind enough to leave a review for this book on Amazon? It'd be greatly appreciated!

Thanks and good luck!

ABOUT THE AUTHOR

Jennifer Sullivan is an accomplished nutritionist, avid researcher, and retains her information like a human encyclopedia! She has been through too much jargon within the diet world to not share it. Her journey has led her to multiple beneficial diet plans that work without a doubt and a couple that are not even worth a mention!

She now tries to convey her trial and error knowledge and vast research by writing ebooks. Jennifer doesn't hesitate to help any and all people she can to discover their true potential through diet so others don't have to go through all the trouble she has.

When not looking into the validity of new up and coming fad diets and diets of yesterday she is enjoying herself with her many free spirited hobbies. Jennifer might be on the beach running, snapping photos of multicolored autumn trees, or even on her bike getting lost on a dirt trail that leads to her next adventure!

Whatever outside experiences Jennifer falls into, she always returns home stat to work on her passion of non fiction writing to add value to the world!

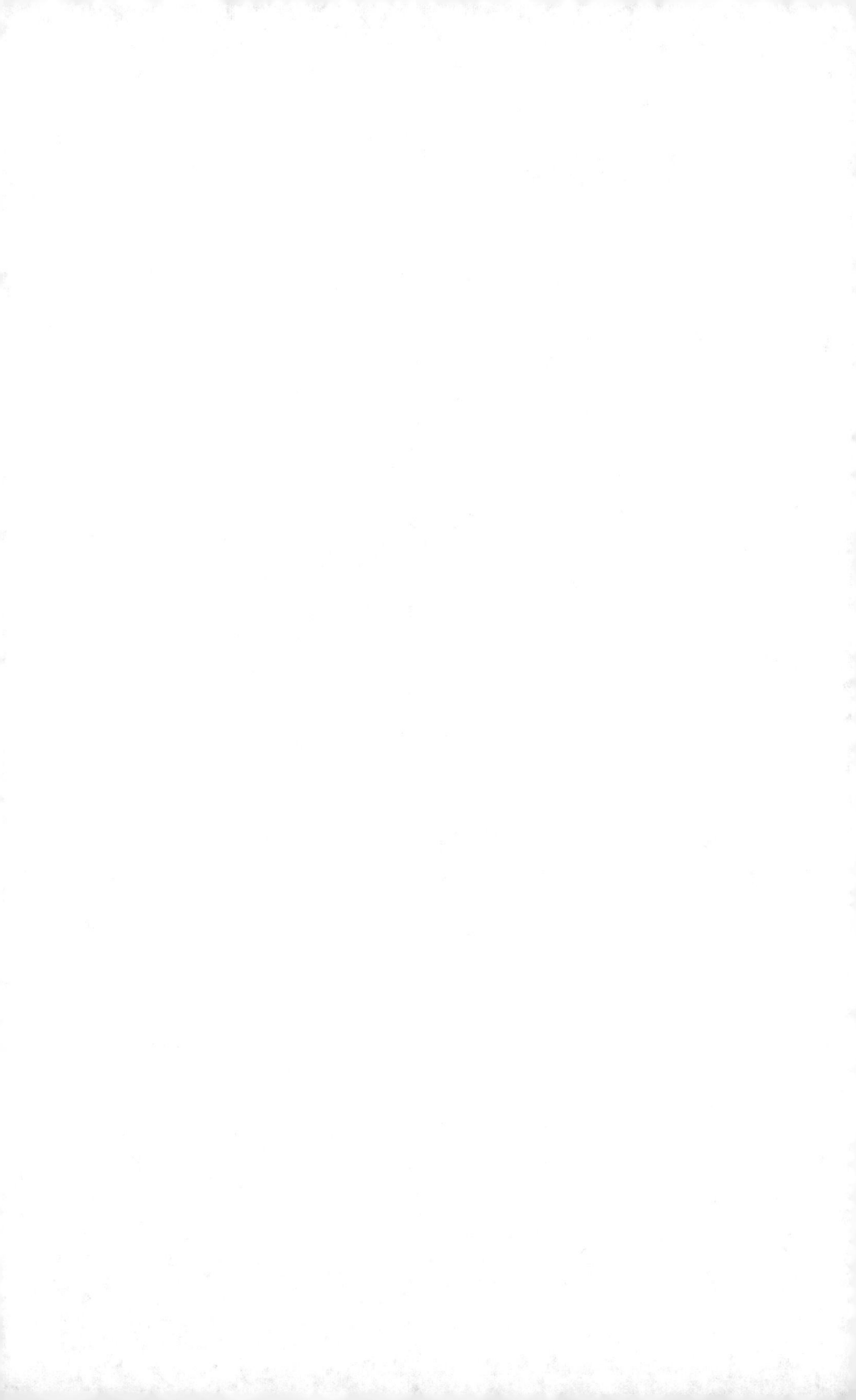

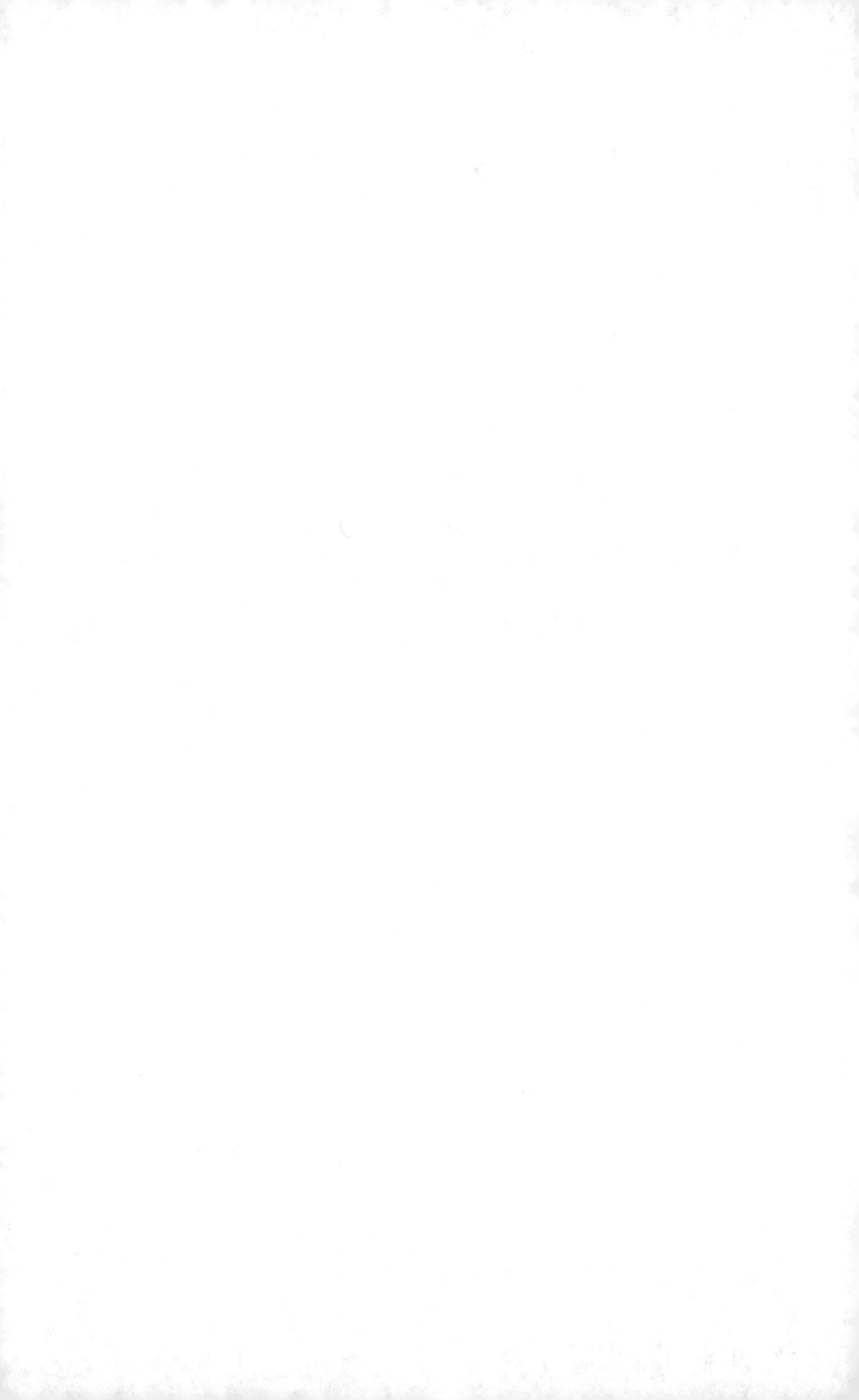

www.ingramcontent.com/pod-product-compliance
Lightning Source LLC
Chambersburg PA
CBHW060224290526
45789CB00003B/1394